I0697067

FERTILITY DIET

FOR NOVICES

Enriched Recipes, Foods, Meal Plan & Procedures That Focuses On Ovulation Improvement, Gaining Knowledge On Fertility Nutrition, Healthy Exercise Plan And More

DR. MATEO GABRIEL

Copyright © [Dr. Mateo Gabriel] [2003]. All rights reserved. You can't copy, distribute, or send any part of this book in any way, including by photocopying, recording, or other electronic or mechanical means, without the publisher's written permission first. The only times this is okay are for short quotes in reviews and other legal noncommercial uses.

DISCLAIMER

The information in this book is only meant to be used for general reading. In any way, the author and publisher do not promise or represent that the information in this work is full, correct, reliable, appropriate, or available. This includes any warranties that are expressed or implied. Because of this, you should only rely on this material at your own risk.

This book is not meant to replace professional help. If you have any questions about a subject, you should always get help from a qualified expert. The author and distributor of this book are not responsible for how the information in it is used or abused.

The author's thoughts and feelings are shown in this book. They do not necessarily represent the official policy or stance of any other person, group, employer, or business.

Any third-party material that you can get to through this book is not endorsed or backed by the author or publisher.

The information in this book is correct at the time it was published, after all possible checks. However, the author and distributor are not responsible for any loss, damage, or inconvenience that may be caused by mistakes or omissions.

TABLE OF CONTENTS

CHAPTER ONE
INTRODUCTION TO FERTILITY DIET

DESCRIBE FERTILITY

The biological term for the capacity of an individual or a couple to conceive and bear children is fertility. When it comes to human reproduction, the ability to conceive a child successfully is frequently used to gauge fertility. A mature egg is released from the ovaries, sperm fertilizes it, and the fertilized egg is then implanted in the uterus in this complex process. Numerous biological, environmental, and lifestyle factors can impact fertility, making it a complex component of human health and reproduction.

VARIABLES IMPACTING FERTILITY

Fertility can be affected by a multitude of circumstances, including external and biological influences. Given that fertility tends to decrease with age, especially in women, age is a critical issue. Over time, changes in the reproductive organs affect the amount and quality of eggs and sperm. Fertility problems can also result from hormonal imbalances, anatomical anomalies, and specific medical disorders. In addition to biological variables, lifestyle decisions like smoking, binge drinking, and being around contaminants can hurt fertility. In addition to these factors, stress and general well-being can also affect reproductive health.

DIET'S IMPACT ON FERTILITY

Fertility is greatly influenced by diet, which is a changeable element that people can improve to increase their chances of becoming pregnant. Diet has a complex effect on fertility that involves both macro- and micronutrients. Reproductive health depends on consuming enough of several key minerals, including zinc, iron, folate, and omega-3 fatty acids. These nutrients aid in the formation of healthy eggs and sperm, regulate hormonal balance, and aid in the implantation of the fertilized egg in the uterus. On the other hand, diets heavy in sugar, trans fats, and processed meals may negatively impact fertility.

A further important component of diet's impact on reproductive health is the correlation between body weight and fertility. The likelihood of pregnancy can be impacted by hormonal imbalances and irregular menstruation, which can arise from being underweight or overweight. Optimizing fertility requires consuming a balanced, nutritious diet to reach and maintain a healthy weight.

CHAPTER TWO

THE FERTILITY DIET'S SCIENTIFIC BASIS

HEALTHY EATING AND REPRODUCTIVE SYSTEMS

In terms of reproductive health, nutrition is essential because it affects both men's and women's fertility. A fertility diet is a specific type of eating plan designed to increase the body's ability to conceive by giving the body the nutrients it needs. Keeping a healthy body weight is important because underweight and obesity can have a detrimental effect on fertility. Reproductive health depends on consuming enough macronutrients (proteins, fats, and carbohydrates) and micronutrients (vitamins and minerals).

DIETARY INFLUENCE ON HORMONAL BALANCE

One of the key factors influencing fertility is how nutrition affects hormone balance. Hormones are essential for controlling both the menstrual cycle and the generation of sperm in women. Deficits or imbalances in some nutrients can upset the delicate hormonal balance, which can result in anovulation, irregular menstrual periods, or decreased sperm production. For instance, insulin resistance, which is frequently linked to a diet high in refined carbs, can impact sex hormone levels and aggravate disorders like PCOS in women.

INVESTIGATIONS AND RESULTS

Numerous investigations have explored the complex connection between reproductive health and nutrition. These investigations frequently look at how particular nutrients or food habits affect the results of conception. Fish and some plant oils contain omega-3 fatty acids, which have been linked to increased fertility in both men and women. Vitamins C and E are examples of antioxidants that help guard against oxidative stress, which can affect the quality of sperm and eggs. Additionally, several studies have connected improved reproductive outcomes to the Mediterranean diet, which is characterized by a high consumption of fruits, vegetables, and whole grains.

The idea of the "fertility window" for women highlights the significance of diet during the time leading up to conception. The developing baby needs to consume enough folate, a B vitamin, before conception and in the early stages of pregnancy to prevent neural tube abnormalities. An additional vital nutrient that helps avoid anemia and supports the increased blood volume during pregnancy is iron. For women who intend to get pregnant, it is essential to make sure their diet is well-balanced and full of a range of nutrient-dense foods.

Dietary variables can affect the quantity and quality of sperm in males. Foods high in zinc, such as meat and nuts, are necessary for the development and operation of sperm. Male fertility and vitamin D, which may be derived from the sun and some meals, have also been related. For males trying to conceive, it is advised to limit their use of soy-based products because they contain components that resemble estrogen and disrupt hormonal balance.

The science underlying the fertility diet examines how nutrition affects reproductive health from a variety of angles. It takes a comprehensive strategy that takes into account both male and female components to fully comprehend the complex interactions between food, hormone balance, and fertility. The guidelines for a fertility-friendly diet are still being shaped by research findings, which highlight the significance of a nutrient-dense, well-balanced diet for supporting the best possible reproductive outcomes.

CHAPTER THREE
EVALUATING YOUR PRESENT DIET

ASSESSMENT OF LIFESTYLE AND FOOD DIARY

Evaluating your present diet entails a thorough investigation of many factors, such as maintaining a food journal and performing a lifestyle assessment. These tools offer insightful information on your general lifestyle choices, nutritional intake, and eating patterns.

A food diary is an organized list of everything you eat within a given time frame, usually a few days or a week. It includes information about portion sizes, timing of meals, and even emotional or contextual elements around your eating habits in addition to just listing the foods. By keeping a food journal, you can get a true understanding of your dietary patterns and pinpoint the advantages and disadvantages of your present eating routine.

When combined with a food diary, a lifestyle assessment takes into account aspects other than food intake. It explores your daily activities, hydration habits, stress levels, sleep patterns, and physical activity. A holistic perspective of your well-being can be obtained by comprehending the connections between your diet and lifestyle choices, which are critical to your entire health. For example, erratic sleep habits or elevated stress levels might affect nutrient absorption and food selection, thus affecting how effective your diet is.

FINDING GAPS IN NUTRIENTS

Finding vitamin gaps is an essential part of evaluating a diet. This entails determining if the amount of important nutrients—such as vitamins, minerals, protein, fats, and carbohydrates—that you currently consume in your diet meets the recommended levels. There is a need to evaluate not only the foods you eat but also the extent to which your body assimilates these nutrients because deficiencies in certain nutrients can result from both inadequate intake and poor absorption.

Comparing nutrient consumption to published dietary standards or recommendations is a frequent method of doing so. These recommendations give standards for the daily or weekly intake of several nutrients according to factors including age, sex, weight, and degree of exercise. You can identify areas that require change by comparing your actual consumption to these suggestions. By identifying any excesses or deficiencies, this procedure helps you make well-informed decisions to maximize your nutrient balance.

It's also essential to comprehend the idea of nutrient density while assessing your diet. Foods that are high in nutrients have a high concentration of vital nutrients about their calorie level. Increasing the amount of foods high in nutrients in your diet guarantees that you get a wide range of vitamins and minerals without ingesting too many calories. This strategy is especially helpful for people who want to improve the nutritional value of their diet without consuming too many high-energy, low-nutrient items.

Evaluating your present diet entails a thorough analysis that extends beyond a list of the foods you consume. A thorough insight into your eating patterns can be obtained by combining a food diary, lifestyle evaluation, and nutrient gap analysis. With this information at hand, you may make well-informed decisions that will maximize your dietary intake and, in turn, your general health and well-being.

CHAPTER FOUR
CRUCIAL ELEMENTS FOR OPTIMAL FERTILITY
VITAMIN FOLIC ACID

A healthy pregnancy and increased fertility are greatly aided by folic acid. This water-soluble B vitamin helps form the neural tube in the early stages of pregnancy and is necessary for DNA synthesis and repair. Adequate consumption of folic acid before conception and throughout the first trimester of pregnancy can considerably lower the growing fetus's risk of neural tube abnormalities. Legumes, fortified cereals, and leafy green vegetables are foods high in folic acid. To guarantee adequate levels, supplements could be advised in some circumstances, especially for women who intend to become pregnant.

THE FATTY ACIDS OMEGA-3

The integrity of the reproductive system depends on omega-3 fatty acids, particularly docosahexaenoic acid (DHA) and eicosapentaenoic acid (EPA). These polyunsaturated lipids, which are especially prevalent in sperm and brain cells, support the structural integrity of cell membranes. Omega-3s can increase both spouses' overall fertility and have been related to better sperm quality in men.

Walnuts, flaxseeds, and fatty fish like salmon and mackerel are good sources of omega-3 fatty acids. Couples looking to maximize their fertility may find it helpful to incorporate these foods into their diet or to think about taking supplements.

OXIDIZERS

The body needs antioxidants to defend against oxidative stress, which can hurt reproductive health. An imbalance between the body's antioxidants and free radicals can lead to oxidative stress, which can harm DNA and cells. Antioxidants that balance this imbalance include vitamin C, vitamin E, and selenium. A wide range of fruits, vegetables, nuts, and seeds contain these chemicals.

Eating a diet high in antioxidants can protect reproductive cells from oxidative damage, which may increase fertility. Couples who are having trouble conceiving may also benefit from taking antioxidant supplements, but it's important to speak with medical professionals before beginning any supplementation.

MINERALS AND VITAMINS

Minerals and vitamins are essential for good health and have a big impact on fertility. For instance, vitamin D insufficiency has been linked to infertility in both men and women. Vitamin D is essential for the control of hormones. Sufficient levels of vitamin D can be achieved by diet, fortified dairy products, and fatty fish, among other things. Adequate exposure to sunlight can also help. Certain minerals, such as iron and zinc, are crucial for maintaining reproductive health.

Iron is necessary to prevent anemia, which can impair menstrual cycles and fertility, while zinc is essential for the growth and motility of sperm. Preserving a diet rich in nutrients and well-balanced with a range of nutrient-dense foods guarantees that the body gets the vitamins and minerals required for maximum fertility.

Furthermore, supplementation under the supervision of medical specialists may be explored to address particular nutrient deficiencies that may impair fertility in circumstances where dietary intake may be inadequate.

CHAPTER FIVE

FORMULATING A MEAL PLAN WITH A FERTILITY FOCUS

MACRONUTRIENT EQUILIBRIUM

Making a meal plan with fertility in mind requires careful consideration of macronutrient balance. Each of the three primary macronutrients fats, proteins, and carbohydrates has a specific function in promoting reproductive health. A balanced consumption of these macronutrients promotes optimal body weight, hormonal balance, and increased fertility. Proteins aid in the development of reproductive tissues, healthy fats are crucial for the generation of hormones, and carbohydrates supply the energy required for biological processes. Maintaining the health of the reproductive system and supporting the body's complex hormonal system depend on striking the correct balance between these macronutrients.

SELECTING FOODS THAT BOOST FERTILITY

A diversified and nutrient-rich diet is essential when selecting meals to increase fertility. Fertility can be improved by including foods high in vitamins, minerals, and antioxidants. Fruits and vegetables are rich in antioxidants, which help fend off oxidative stress, which can be harmful to reproductive health. Legumes and other foods high in folate are important for fetal development and can help prevent neural tube abnormalities. Flaxseeds and fatty fish are good sources of omega-3 fatty acids, which help maintain hormonal balance and a healthy reproductive system. A meal plan that includes a variety of nutrient-dense foods guarantees that the body gets a wide range of vital nutrients that are beneficial to fertility.

TIPS FOR MEAL PLANNING

The goal of meal planning advice for fertility should be to create a sustainable and well-rounded approach to nutrition.

It's crucial to be consistent and to continue consuming the same amount of nutrients throughout the day. Adding a range of vibrant fruits and vegetables to meals not only improves their presentation but also supplies essential vitamins and minerals for healthy reproduction. Selecting whole grains instead of processed grains helps control blood sugar levels, which are good for hormonal balance and guarantees a consistent release of energy. Lean protein consumption, derived from fish, poultry, and plant-based foods, promotes muscular health and supplies vital amino acids for reproductive tissues.

In addition, as being underweight or overweight can affect fertility, controlling portion sizes is essential to maintaining a healthy weight. Though sometimes disregarded, enough hydration is essential for maintaining general health, which includes reproductive health. Maintaining proper hydration promotes all-around health, including the generation of cervical mucus, which is important for conception. Limiting processed foods, sugary drinks, and too much caffeine is also advised because these can have a bad impact on reproductive health and hormone balance.

A meal plan with an emphasis on fertility should carefully balance macronutrients, include foods that increase fertility, and follow smart meal planning advice. A balanced diet consisting of carbohydrates, proteins, and fats can help people conceive more easily and promote reproductive health. Nutrient-dense, whole foods should be prioritized. The integration of a comprehensive strategy for promoting fertility and overall well-being with lifestyle aspects like portion control and hydration is enhanced by the holistic approach to meal planning.

CHAPTER SIX
RECIPES FOR STUNTING
BREAKFAST CONCEPTS

A healthy, balanced breakfast is essential for promoting fertility. Including complete foods high in vital nutrients can have a beneficial effect on reproductive health. Think about having a large dish of oats with nuts and fresh fruit on top to start your day. Oatmeal is a great source of fiber and complex carbs that help control blood sugar levels. Berries are one of the foods that add flavor and a good source of antioxidants.

Eggs are yet another breakfast option that promotes fertility. They include essential nutrients including chlorine, which is connected to the development of the fetus's brain, and are an excellent source of high-quality protein. In addition to being delicious, scrambled eggs with spinach and tomatoes provide a variety of vitamins and minerals that are good for fertility.

Including items that increase fertility, such as avocados, in your breakfast can supply important healthy fats. For extra nutritional value, try spreading avocado on whole-grain toast and adding sesame seeds on top. In addition to promoting reproductive health, this combo gives you steady energy throughout the morning.

RECIPES FOR LUNCH AND DINNER

Make sure your lunch and dinner are well-rounded meals with a range of nutrient-dense foods. Because grilled salmon is high in omega-3 fatty acids, it's a great option to promote conception. For a well-balanced meal that includes protein, fiber, and important vitamins, serve it with quinoa and steamed vegetables.

A lentil and vegetable stew served over brown rice is one example of a vegetarian dish. The fiber in brown rice lowers blood sugar levels, while lentils are an excellent source of plant-based protein. Adding vibrant veggies like spinach and bell peppers gives the dish a range of antioxidants in addition to improving its aesthetic appeal.

Include whole grains in your lunch and supper meals, such as barley or farro. Fiber from these grains promotes healthy digestion and balances hormones. A tasty and fertility-friendly option would be to make a colorful stir-fry with tofu and a variety of vegetables.

SMOOTHIES AND SNACKS

Selecting the appropriate snacks can be quite important for sustaining energy and promoting conception. Choose a handful of nuts, like walnuts or almonds, as they are high in vital nutrients and healthy fats. Another great snack is Greek yogurt with berries, which provides antioxidants, probiotics, and protein.

Smoothies are a tasty and easy way to include foods in your diet that increase fertility. Blend items such as spinach, pineapple, and banana to make a fertility smoothie.

While pineapple has a natural sweetness and can have anti-inflammatory qualities, spinach contributes folate. To boost the protein content of the smoothie, add a scoop of protein powder.

Concentrating on a diet rich in nutrients that is well-rounded and contains a range of nutrient-dense foods can support reproductive health in general. Fertility-friendly items can be added to smoothies, breakfast, lunch, supper, snacks, and other meals to help support fertility and improve overall health.

CHAPTER SEVEN
LIFESTYLE ELEMENTS
FERTILITY AND EXERCISE

In addition to being vital for preserving general health, regular physical activity has recently drawn attention for its impact on fertility. Moderate physical activity has been linked to beneficial outcomes for reproductive health. Exercise aids in the regulation of hormones that affect fertility, including cortisol and insulin. Furthermore, consistent physical exercise that maintains a healthy weight is associated with better reproductive outcomes. But it's important to find a balance because too much exercise, particularly severe training, can negatively impact a person's ability to conceive in both men and women.

PHYSICAL ACTIVITY'S EFFECT

Engaging in physical activity improves general well-being and helps one maintain a healthy weight. It has a good impact on several physiological functions, such as blood circulation, which may indirectly improve reproductive health. Exercise regularly has been demonstrated to lower the risk of diseases like polycystic ovarian syndrome (PCOS), which is a prevalent cause of infertility in women. Physically active men can maintain optimal sperm motility and production. Harnessing the benefits of physical activity on fertility requires finding a balance between maintaining an active lifestyle and abstaining from excessive exercise.

FERTILITY-FRIENDLY EXERCISE PLANS

Selecting workouts that promote fertility entails designing fitness regimens that assist with reproductive health. Walking, swimming, and mild yoga are examples of low-impact exercises that are frequently advised for those who are trying to get pregnant. These workouts reduce the danger of harm and stress on the reproductive organs in addition to improving cardiovascular health. However, adding strength training can be advantageous for both sexes since it improves general fitness and aids in preserving a good body composition, both of which are critical for fertility.

HANDLING STRESS TO CONCEIVE

It has been determined that stress may have an impact on fertility, thus controlling it is crucial for individuals trying to get pregnant. Persistent stress can throw off the hormonal balance, affecting sperm production in men and causing irregular menstrual cycles in women. Although complete stress elimination is unattainable, the negative effects of stress on fertility can be lessened by implementing stress-reduction techniques. Managing stress during the conception process requires practicing mindfulness, setting up a supportive atmosphere, and getting expert assistance when necessary.

THE IMPACT OF STRESS ON FERTILITY

There is ample evidence to support the complex relationship between stress and fertility. The reproductive system can be impacted by high amounts of stress because they can cause the release of stress hormones like cortisol, which can upset the delicate hormonal balance required for conception. Stress can lead to anovulation, irregular menstrual periods, and even failed implantations in women. Stress can alter the quantity and quality of sperm in men. Couples navigating the reproductive process must identify their stressors and put stress-reduction strategies into practice.

UNWINDING METHODS

Including relaxation methods in daily life can be a beneficial approach to promoting conception. By triggering the body's relaxation response, methods including progressive muscle relaxation, deep breathing, and meditation help mitigate the negative consequences of stress. Mind-body exercises, such as tai chi and yoga, not only enhance physical health but also create a mental space for rest. By lowering stress levels and promoting a healthier body and mind, including these strategies in a routine can help establish a favorable environment for conception.

CHAPTER EIGHT

PARTICULAR POINTS TO REMEMBER

MALE FERTILITY DIET

For men to maximize their reproductive health and increase their chances of conception, a fertility diet is essential. It highlights how crucial a healthy, well-balanced diet is to boosting both the quality and quantity of sperm. A fertility diet should contain sufficient amounts of vitamins, minerals, antioxidants, and vital fatty acids. Sperm health is enhanced by diets high in zinc, selenium, vitamin C, and omega-3 fatty acids. A crucial component of a male fertility-focused diet is also keeping a healthy weight and limiting alcohol and caffeine intake.

MEN'S HEALTH AND REPRODUCTION

The term "male reproductive health" refers to a variety of variables that affect both general health and fertility. The motility, quality, and quantity of sperm are essential elements of male reproductive health. Male fertility can be impacted by underlying medical issues, environmental exposures, lifestyle decisions, and other factors. Men can maintain good reproductive health by controlling stress, eating a balanced diet, and exercising regularly. People who want to increase their fertility must get medical advice as soon as possible to address any possible problems.

FOODS AND MINERALS THAT PROMOTE SPERM HEALTH

Nutrients and diets that are specific to sperm health are important. Fruits and vegetables are rich in antioxidants, which help prevent oxidative stress and can lower the quality of sperm. Nuts and seeds are rich sources of zinc, which is necessary for sperm development and function. Sperm membrane integrity is aided by omega-3 fatty acids, which are frequently present in fish. Getting your vitamin D from pills or sunshine exposure is linked to increased sperm motility. Sperm health can be improved with a diet high in certain nutrients and a healthy lifestyle.

TAKING CARE OF TYPICAL FERTILITY PROBLEMS

Common problems that can impair a couple's capacity to conceive are frequently faced by couples dealing with fertility difficulties. To find any contributing factors, a thorough fertility evaluation should be performed on both couples. Essential first actions include addressing lifestyle variables such as excessive alcohol intake, smoking, and keeping a healthy body weight. Based on the particular concerns found, prompt medical intervention, including fertility treatments, might be required. Throughout the reproductive process, spouses and medical experts must have open lines of communication, offer emotional support, and work together.

PCOS, OR POLYCYSTIC OVARIAN SYNDROME

PCOS, or polycystic ovarian syndrome, is a prevalent endocrine illness that primarily affects women and people of reproductive age. Ovarian cysts, irregular menstrual cycles, and high testosterone levels are its defining features. PCOS can affect ovulation, which might affect fertility. Lifestyle changes like maintaining a healthy weight, getting regular exercise, and eating a balanced diet are common management techniques. Additionally, doctors may prescribe medication to enhance ovulation and control menstrual periods. To treat the complex interplay of factors related to PCOS, individuals may benefit from a multidisciplinary approach comprising gynecologists, endocrinologists, and nutritionists.

DIABETOMYCOSIS

A disorder known as endometriosis occurs when tissue that resembles the lining of the uterus grows outside of it. This may impair fertility by causing discomfort, irritation, and adhesion development. Endometriosis can be treated with medication, surgery, or a combination of the two. The goal of fertility-preserving surgery is to protect reproductive organs while removing endometriotic lesions. In addition, couples experiencing infertility as a result of endometriosis may be advised to consider assisted reproductive technologies (ART), such as in vitro fertilization (IVF).

UNKNOWN CAUSE OF INFERTILITY

Couples with comprehensive fertility examinations that reveal no obvious problems yet are still unable to conceive are diagnosed with unexplained infertility, a difficult diagnosis. It highlights the intricacy of reproductive health and the boundaries of present medical knowledge. A combination of lifestyle modifications, psychological support, and different reproductive therapies are used to manage infertility that cannot be explained. When other treatments fail, assisted reproductive technologies like IVF may be taken into consideration. Navigating the uncertainty connected with infertility that doesn't seem to make sense requires maintaining open communication with medical specialists and providing emotional support within the partnership.

CHAPTER NINE

MONITORING MENSTRUAL AND OVULATION CYCLES

KNOWLEDGE OF THE MENSTRUAL CYCLE

In women of reproductive age, the menstrual cycle is a complicated and detailed biological process. It is usually broken up into several parts and lasts approximately 28 days, however, there are often variances. If there has been no pregnancy, the menstrual cycle starts with menstruation, which is the shedding of the uterine lining. The follicular phase then starts as the body gets ready for ovulation. Follicle-stimulating hormone (FSH) stimulates the ovary to produce a follicle that contains an egg at this period. The follicle produces estrogen as it ages, which causes the uterine lining to thicken in anticipation of a possible pregnancy.

METHODS FOR PREDICTING OVULATION

For people who want to get pregnant or who want to prevent getting pregnant, being able to predict ovulation accurately is essential. Ovulation tracking can be done in several ways, from the more conventional calendar method to more sophisticated procedures. Using the calendar technique, patterns can be found and fertile days can be predicted by tracking the menstrual cycle over several months. Monitoring basal body temperature (BBT), where a modest increase in temperature signifies ovulation, is an additional strategy. Furthermore, tracking alterations in cervical mucus offers insightful information about fertility. Ovulation prediction kits, which identify the spike in luteinizing hormone (LH) before ovulation, are examples of advanced techniques.

LOOKING FOR EXPERT ADVICE

Seeking expert assistance is essential for folks who are having trouble getting pregnant or who have irregular menstrual periods. Reproductive endocrinologists and gynecologists are two medical professionals to speak with to determine the root causes of problems impacting fertility. These experts can carry out comprehensive examinations, such as hormone assessments and imaging studies, to identify any potential barriers to conception. By consulting an expert, people can receive customized recommendations that are suited to their unique situation, increasing the likelihood of a successful conception.

WHEN TO SEE A SPECIALIST IN FERTILITY

While many couples will be able to conceive naturally, some may face challenges. If frequent, unprotected sexual activity does not result in conception within a year for women under 35, or within six months for women 35 and beyond, the standard recommendation is to see a fertility expert. Furthermore, people with pre-existing medical disorders or recognized reproductive health issues ought to seek professional advice sooner rather than later. If required, fertility specialists can assist couples with assisted reproductive technologies, recommend suitable procedures, and perform thorough examinations.

UTILIZING A NUTRITIONIST

Nutrition affects hormone balance and general health, which is important for reproductive health. For those who want to maximize their fertility, working with a dietitian can be helpful. A nutritionist can offer tailored dietary advice, guaranteeing sufficient consumption of vital nutrients that promote reproductive health. It's crucial to maintain a healthy weight through diet because weight extremes, whether underweight or overweight, might affect fertility. A nutritionist can collaborate with medical professionals to develop a comprehensive strategy that takes medical and nutritional factors into account, promoting an environment that is favorable to successful reproduction.

www.ingramcontent.com/pod-product-compliance
Lightning Source LLC
Chambersburg PA
CBHW060805260726

48660CB00002B/789